Immunomodulators in oral diseases

Farzhana T H
Prashanth Shenoy
Laxmikanth Chatra

Immunomodulators in oral diseases

LAP LAMBERT Academic Publishing

Imprint

Any brand names and product names mentioned in this book are subject to trademark, brand or patent protection and are trademarks or registered trademarks of their respective holders. The use of brand names, product names, common names, trade names, product descriptions etc. even without a particular marking in this work is in no way to be construed to mean that such names may be regarded as unrestricted in respect of trademark and brand protection legislation and could thus be used by anyone.

Cover image: www.ingimage.com

Publisher:
LAP LAMBERT Academic Publishing
is a trademark of
International Book Market Service Ltd., member of OmniScriptum Publishing Group
17 Meldrum Street, Beau Bassin 71504, Mauritius

Printed at: see last page
ISBN: 978-620-0-09990-7

Zugl. / Approved by: Mangalore, Yenepoya University,2019

Table of Contents

INTRODUCTION

The oral cavity is a universe of various numerous diseases, which may be developmental, infective, inflammatory and immunological etc. Immunology plays a very important role in homeostasis but it possesses two edge sword actions.

Immunology is one of the most rapidly rising area of medical biotechnology research and has great promises with regard to the prevention and treatment of a wide range of disorders such as the inflammatory diseases of skin, gut, respiratory tract, joints and central organs. In addition infectious diseases are now primarily considered immunological disorders while neoplastic diseases, organ transplantation and several autoimmune diseases may involve in an immunosuppressive state[1]. The immune system is one of our most complex biological systems in the body. The basic role of the immune system is to distinguish self from non-self [2].

Immune system is a system of biological structures and processes within an organism that protects against disease. To function properly, an immune system must detect a wide variety of agents, from viruses to parasitic worms, and distinguish them from the organism's own healthy tissue. The immune system recognizes foreign bodies and responds with the production of immune cells and proteins.Barriers help an organism to defend itself from the many dangerous pathogens it may encounter. Barrier defenses include the skin and mucous membranes of the respiratory, urinary, and reproductive tracts.Mucus traps and allows for the removal of microbes as m any body fluids including saliva, mucus, and tears are hostile to microbes.

The term immunity means the resistance exhibited by the host towards injury caused by microorganisms and their products (toxins). This is based on the property of self and non self recognition. That means immunity is carried out by the process of recognition and disposal of non self or materials that enter the body. Immune response is the reaction of the body against any foreign antigen. But protection against infection disease is only a part of it. Immunity is of two types namely innate and acquired immunity.1. Innate (or natural or non-specific) and 2. Adaptive (or acquired or specific) [3]. Both these responses have two components each, that is, cellular and humoral. As there is no involvement of memory cells Innate immunity lacks specificity. Acquired immunity on other hand is specifically adapted for the inducing pathogens and due to the presence of memory cell line, response improves with subsequent exposures to the same pathogen. In the innate cellular immunity there is involvement of monocytesmacrophage system, while in innate humoral immunity there is activation of component system. On the other hand the cellular component of acquired immunity involves of T-lymphocytes while the humoral component of this immunity involves the role of Blymphocytes. Normally in innate and acquired immune responses act in combined manner to contain or eradicate infection. In some cases innate responses are enough to deactivate the offending agent. However in many other cases, certain cells of innate immune system, such as antigen presenting cells (APC), can also process the offending agent into smaller fragments which then activate adaptive immune system to deactivate or kill these pathogens. The elements which are formed in the blood include erythrocytes (RBC), leukocytes (WBC) and thrombocytes (platelets). The leukocytes are of two types: granulocytes (neutrophils, eosinophils and basophils cells) and agranulocytes (T-lymphocytes, Blymphocytes and monocytes). The process by which blood cells are formed is called as haemopoiesis. All such cells are involved in exerting immune response develops from pluripotent haemotopoietic stem cells which is present in bone marrow. These stem cell gives rise to lymphoid stem cell, trilineage myeloid stem cell, megakaryocytes (from platelets) and erythroblasts (from erythrocytes). The lymphoid stem cells through their progenitors, gives rise to mature lymphocytes (T-lymphocytes and Blymphocytes) and natural killer cells (NK cells). T- and Blymphocytes are involved in mediating adaptive immune responses while NK cells exert innate immune response along with mature cells originating from trilineage myeloid stem cells. When exposed to specific antigens, B-lymphocytes differentiate into antibody producing plasma cells in the bone marrow. Simultaneously, t-cells, under the influence of thymic hormones, migrate to the thymus and on appropriate stimulus by antigen presenting cells (APC) acquire T-cell receptor (TCR) and get differentiated to helper T-cells (with specific protein cluster of differentiation- CD4+) and cytotoxic T-cells (with specific protein cluster of differentiation- CD8+). The CD4+ (TH cell) subtypes of T-cells differentiate further outside the thymus into several phenotypes: TH1, TH2 and TH3 which are distinguished by the different cytokines (IL-2 and IFN-γ) they synthesize. TH1 T-cells produce cytokines that stimulate proliferation and differentiation of T-lymphocytes and NK cells. These cytokine play an important role in cell mediated immunity (CMI). TG2 T-cells release cytokine (IL-4, IL-5, IL-10 and IL-13) that stimulate B-lymphocytes production for humoral immunity. TH3 T-cells play an important role in resting phases of immune response and in the production of anti-inflammatory immunoglobin-A (iga) antibodies that are important in secretory immunity [4].

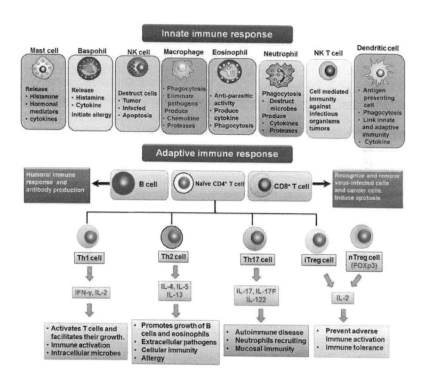

There are a several immunological diseases affecting the oral cavity those have involve pathogenesis. In these cases, steroid is the mainstay, but steroid has their own deleterious side effect when utilized for longer time and even sometime steroid is not enough alone to remedy disease due to involute pathogenic factors and some disease can be steroid resistant. In these cases, immunomodulatory drugs should be administered.Immuno Refers to immune response, immune system, and modulation is the act of modifying according to due measure and proportion. Thus, immunomodulators are natural or synthetic substances that help to regulate or normalize the immune system.[5] The benefits of immunomodulators is their ability to stimulate natural and adaptive defense mechanisms, such as cytokines, which enables the body to help itself.[6] Immunomodulators modulate the immune reaction and reduce inflammatory replication. An immunomodulators should be given along with a steroid to spare side effect and speed the rejuvenating process. For these reasons these drugs come under the category of —steroid sparing drugs. Utilization of immunomodulators reduce the dose of steroid, decrease the chances of the deleterious effect of steroid and increasethe rejuvenating time. These drugs can be given alone too in certain circumstances like very astringent cases and cases non-respondent to steroids.

The natural immunomodulators act to strengthen weak immune systems and to moderate immune systems that are overactive. Plant sterols and sterolins are natural immunomodulators found in some raw fruits and vegetables and in the alga, spirulina. Spreads and yoghurt type foods containing high levels of plant sterols are commonly to be found on sale as 'cholesterol-reducing' agents. These compounds are destroyed when vegetables and fruits are cooked. Other natural immunomodulators include aloe vera, plumbago indica, aegle marmalos. [7]ginseng root, chamomile tea, reishi mushroom extract, olive leaf extract, N. Sativa oil, polysaccharides isolated from Juniperus scopolorum, ficus carica leaf extract, Isodon serra extract.[1,8,9,10,] In children, immunomodulators are less likely to cause growth failure than corticosteroids. Topical immunomodulators are well tolerated even in infants. [11]

IMMUNOMODULATORS

IMMUNOMODULATION:

Immunomodulation is a therapeutic approach in which try to intervene in auto regulating processes of the defense system. Immunomodulator are the intrnsic or extrinsic substances which regulate or alter the scope type duration or competency of the immune response. Immunomodulator correct immune system that is out of balance. Immunomodulators modulate the activity of the immune system. That, in turn reduces the inflammatory response. Hence, immunomodulator is to maintain a disease Free State & modulation of immune response by suppression and stimulation. Immunomodulator can give supportive therapy to the chemotherapy. Immunomodulator are natural or synthetic substances which helps to regulate or normalize the immune system. Natural immunomodulator are less potent then prescription immunomodulator and also less likely to cause side effects. Synthetic immunomodulator medication works by suppressing the immune system[12]

Immunomodulator stem from their ability to stimulate natural and adaptive defence mechanism which enables the body to help itself. Natural immunomodulator found in some raw fruits and vegetables and in the alga, sprulina, Aloe vera, Plumbago indica and Aegle marmalose ginseng root, chamomile tea, reishi mushroom extract, olive leaf extract, N. Sativa oil, polysaccharides isolated from Juniperus scopolorum, ficus carica leaf extract, Isodon serra extract etc. [1,8,9,10,12]

Immunomodulatory drugs are divided into two main categories, are- Immunosuppressant and Immunostimulants.[5]

Conditions where immunomodulatory drugs should be advised[5,13]:

- When no response to corticosteroids
- The cases where corticosteroids are contraindicated
- Cases resistant to steroids
- Recurrent cases
- Cases with the previous history of severe adverse effect with steroids.
- No respond to aminosalicylates, antibiotics or corticosteroids.
- Steroid-dependent disease or frequently required steroids.
- Experienced side effects with corticosteroid treatment.
- Perennial disease that does not respond to antibiotics.
- Fistulas (abnormal channels between two loops of intestine or between the intestine and another structure).
- A need to maintain remission.

There are two type of immunomodulators. These can either function as:

1. Immunosuppressants

2. Immunostimulants.

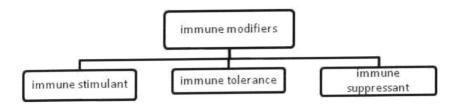

Immunosuppressants

An immunosuppressant is any substance which performs immunosuppression of the immune system. They may be either exogenous, as immunosuppressive drugs, or endogenous, as e.g., testosterone. Immunosuppressants are the agent which suppress the immune system and are used for the control of pathological response in autoimmune disease. The term immunotoxin is also sometimes used to label undesirable immunosuppressants, such as various pollutants and the herbicide DDT are immunosuppressant. [14]

Immune tolerance: Immune tolerance or immunological tolerance is the process by which the immune system does not attack an antigen.It can be either 'natural' or 'self-tolerance', in which the body does not mount an immune response to self-antigens, or 'induced tolerance', in which tolerance to external antigens can be created by manipulating the immune system[12].

Immunostimulants:

Immunostimulants, also known as immunostimulators, are substances (drugs and nutrients) that stimulate the immune system by inducing activation or increasing activity of any of its components. One notable example is the granulocyte macrophage colony-stimulating factor. An immune disorder such as immunodeficiency state autoimmune disease cancer and viral infection can be treated with immunostimulant drug. Fig. 1 shows that the how many types immune system present in human body and how it works to stable our body against foreign particle [15].

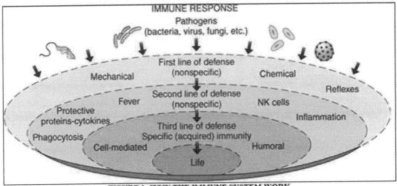

FIGURE 1: HOW THE IMMUNE SYSTEM WORK

There are two main categories of immunostimulators:

Specific immunostimulators

These drugs provide the antigenic specificity in immune response, such as vaccines or any antigen.

Non-specific immunostimulators

These are the agents irrespective of antigenic specificity, augment immune response of other antigen or stimulate components of the immune system without antigenic specificity, such as adjuvant and non-specific immunostimulators. Many endogenous substances are non-specific immunostimulators. For example, female sex hormones are known to stimulate both adaptive and innate immune responses. Some autoimmune diseases such as lupus erythematosus strike women preferentially, and their onset often coincides with puberty. Other hormones appear to regulate the immune system as well, most notably prolactin, growth hormone and vitamin D[43].

Apart from this there are many natural /herbal immunomodulators which strengthen weak immune systems and to moderate immune systems that are overactive.[1,28]

IMMUNOMODULATORY DRUGS

All drugs which modify immune response generally categorized as immunomodulators. These can either function as:

1. Immunosuppressants

2. Immunostimulants.

Some of these can have both the properties depending on which component of immune response they affect. There is also an upcoming generation of immunosuppressants called tolerogens.

IMMUNOSUPPRESSANTS

Drugs which are used to suppress the immunity are called immunonomodulatory drugs.Since, immunity confers resistance to disease, the use of drugs for deliberately suppressing it appears odd at first sight. However, according to the present concept, the ability of the body to recognize self from nonself or foreign, which is the basis of immunity, is liable to cause disorders due to failure to recognize and tolerate antigens produced by its own tissues.[13]

MECHANISM OF ACTION OF IMMUNOSUPPRESSIVE DRUG

Generation of humoral and cell-mediated immune response and sites of action of immunosuppressant drugs.The antigen (Ag) is processed by macrophages or other antigen presenting cells (APC), coupled with class II major histocompatibility complex (MHC) and presented to the CD4 helper cell which are activated by interleukin-I (IL-I), proliferate and secrete cytokines—these in turn promote proliferation and differentiation of antigen activated B cells into antibody (Ab) secreting plasma cells. Antibodies finally bind and inactivate the antigen.

In cell-mediated immunity—foreign antigen is processed and presented to CD4 helper T cells which elaborate IL-2 and other cytokines that in turn stimulate proliferation and maturation of precursor cytotoxic lymphocytes (CTL) that have been activated by antigen presented with class I MHC. The mature CTL (Killer cells) recognize cells carrying the antigen and lyse them.

1. Glucocorticoids inhibit MHC expression and IL-1, IL-2, IL-6 production so that helper T cells are not activated.

2. Cytotoxic drugs block proliferation and differentiation of T and B cells.

3.   Cyclosporine and tacrolimus inhibit antigen stimulated activation and proliferation of helper T cells as well as expression of IL-2 and other cytokines by them.

Antibodies like muromonab CD3, antithymocyte globulin specific bind to helper T cells, prevent their response and deplete them

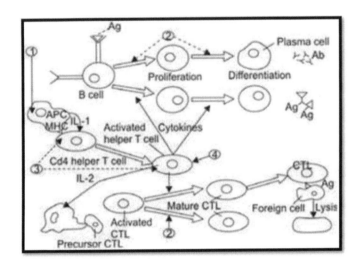

Mechanism of action of immunosuppressive drugs

(Courtesy: Tripathi KD: Essentials of Dental Pharmacology; 305)

CLASSIFICATION IMMUNOSUPPRESSANT S

According to Patil US et al 2012[1]

I. Inhibitors of Lymphocyte Gene Expression
- Glucocorticoids

II. Inhibitors of Lymphocyte Signaling
   a) Calcineurin Inhibitors
   - Cyclosporine
   - Tacrolimus
   b) Mtor Inhibitors
   - Sirolimus
   - Everolimus

III. Cytotoxic Agents

   A) Antimetabolites

   - Azathiprine
   - Mthotrexate
   - Leflunomid.

   B)Alkylating agents

   - Cyclophosphamide

IV. Cytokine Inhibitors
   a) TNF-α Inhibitors
   - Etanercept
   - Infliximab

- Adalimumab

b)   IL-1 Inhibitors

- Anakinra

c)   IL-2 Inhibtors

- Daclizumab

- Basiliximab

V. Antibodies against Specific Immune Cell Molecules

    a)   Polyclonal Antibodies

    - Antithymocyte Globulin (ATG)

    b)   Monoclonal Antibodies

    - Alemutuzmab

    - Muromunab

VI. Inhibitors of Immune Cell Adhesion

    - Efalizumab (LFA-1 Inhibitor)

VII. Miscellaneous

    - Rho (D) Immune Globulin

According to Pagare SS et al[13]

I. Those which act by general suppression of all immune responses

    i)   Antimetabolites

    - Azathioprine

    - Methotrexate

    - Cyclophosphamide

    - Chlorambucil

ii)   Nucleotide synthesis inhibitors

- Mycophenolate mofetil
- Leflunomide

II. Those which are specific suppressants of certain immune responses

- Antilymphocytic serum (ALS)
- Cyclosporine,tacrolimus
- Sirolimus

III. Highly selective monoclonal antibodies

i. Depleting antibodies (against T cells, B cells or both)

- Muromonab
- Rituximab
- Antithymocyte globulin.

ii. Non-depleting antibodies and fusion proteins

- Daclizumab
- Basiliximab

IV. Those which reduce the unwanted reactions due to immune responses, by their antiinflammatory actions

I   Glucocorticoids

- Prednisolone
- Thalidomide

CHOOSING IMMUNOSUPPRESSIVE REGIMENS[86]

In order to make sound judgements when choosing a treatment protocol the clinician has to consider the clinical trial evidence and then decide:

Is the aim to pre-empt an anticipated immune response or to suppress an established immune-mediated inflammation

- In the case of an immune disease, how much immunosuppression will be required and for how long (that is, an assessment of disease activity)? Consider:
  - The natural history of the untreated disease
  - Is the disease multiphasic or 'single shot'
  - The extent and severity of the disease in this particular patient
  - Is the affected organ beyond recovery?
  - The likelihood of relapse
  - The ability to monitor disease parameters long term
- Is this patient likely to withstand the treatment recommended (host fitness parameters)? Consider:
  - Age (older patients are easier to immunosuppress but have a greater risk of infection)
  - Sepsis risk
  - Cancer risk
  - Cardiovascular/diabetes risk
  - Presence of comorbidities
  - Patient compliance and availability for follow-up.
- In choosing the dose and duration of immunosuppressive treatments, one must always weigh disease activity versus host fitness.

IMMUNOSUPPPRESSANTS

CORTICOSTEROIDS

Corticosteroids are natural hormone released by adrenal cortex. These hormone have different role specially antiinflammatory and immunosuppressive action, which are important to cure the oral disease. Its synthetic analogues are given in the form of the drug to cure multiple inflammatory and immunomodulatory drugs. Mechanism of action: Inhibition of migration of leukocytes, Decrease the production of endothelial leukocyte adhesion molecule(ELAM) and ICAM in endothelial cell so the adhesion and localization is decreased, Decrease the chemotaxis, Inhibition of phagocytosis, Stabilization of membranes of the intracellular lysozyme, which contains hydrolytic enzymes so Inhibition of lysozyme release from granulocyte, Release of anti-inflammatory molecules such as lipocortin-1, interleukins IL-10, IL-1ra, and nuclear factor-B, by macrophages, eosinophils, lymphocytes, dendritic cells, neutrophils, and endothelial and epithelial cells, Induction of lipocortins in macrophage, endothelium, fibroblast which inhibit phospholipase A2 and decrease PG, Decrease production of IL1, 2, 3, 6, TNF-α, GM-CSF, Interferon, induce the transcription of the gene encoding the inhibitor of Nuclear Factor Kappa B subtype a (ikba), which reduces the amount of NF-B that translocates to the nucleus and the secretion of pro-inflammatory cytokines and Suppress T cells by decreasing the number of circulating T lymphocytes.

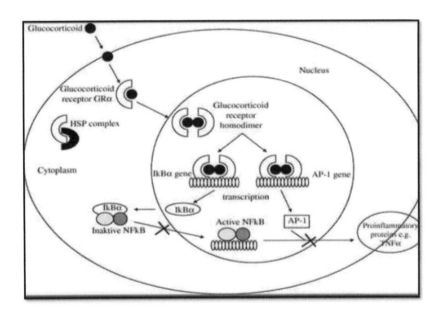

INDICATION:

Oral indication these are mainly based on immunomodulatory action are: Oral Lichen Planus, Oral submucous fibrosis, Aphthous stomatitis, Pemphigus, Pemphigoid, Erythema multiforme, Epidermolysis bullosa, Behcet's Disease, Orofacial Granulomatosis, Sjogren syndrome.[16-27]

- **Lichen planus**
  - Topical Corticosteroids
  > Drug of choice 0.05% clobetasol propionate, 0.1 %Triamcinolone acetonide, 0.05%fluocinonide0.1%, fluocinolone acetonide
  > Apply 2-3 times/day for 3 weeks, followed by tapering during the following 9 weeks
  - Intralesional Corticosteroids

➢ Used tomanage persistent localized lesion and lesions unresponsive to topical therapy.

➢ 10-20mg of insoluble Triamcinolone acetonide is diluted with 0.5ml saline or 2%lidocaine injected to lesion which solubilize gradually 3-4 times/week or 2 times/week

▪ Systemic Corticosteroids

➢ Should be administered only in recalcitrant lesions

➢ 1mg/kg body weight for 7 days, followed by a reduction of 10 mg each subsequent day.

- **Oral submucous fibrosis**

➢ Although it is a chronic inflammatory disease, immunological features had been discovered. Intralesional submucosal injections of a combination of dexamethasone (4 mg/ml) and two parts of hyaluronidase (1500IU) diluted in 1.0 ml of 2% xylocaine twice a week.

- **Recurrent Aphthous stomatitis**

▪ Topical corticosteroids

➢ Topical corticosteroids should be advised in moderate cases where primary methods have been failed.

➢ Topical agents are Dexamethasone 0.05 mg/ml rinsing three times a day, Dexamethasone 0.05 mg/ml with 0.2% chlorhexidine mouthwash for rinsing thrice a day, Clobetasol ointment 0.05% in orabase (1:1), Fluocinonide ointment 0.05% in orabase (1:1) three times a day, Triamcinolone acetonide 0.1% oral paste.

▪ Systemic corticosteroid therapy

➢ Recommended for patients with recalcitrant cases

➢ Hydrocortisone 20 mg or triamcinolone 4 mg, Prednisolone (10-30mg/day) for 10-15 days.

- **Pemphigus**

- Prednisolone doses of 40–60 mg /day for mild case and 60–100 mg/ day in severe case for about 6–8 weeks.If there is no response within 5–7 days, the dose should be increased in 50–100% increments until there is disease control.

- If doses above 100 mg/ day are required, pulsed intravenous CS could be considered.

- **Mucous Membrane Pemphigoid**

  ▪ Topical drugs

  ➢ Fluocinonide 0.05% or clobetasol propionate 0.05% in an adhesive thrice daily for 9–24 weeks).Triamcinolone acetonide can be used intralesionally (in a dilution of 5.0–10 mg/ml) to treat isolated erosions.

  ▪ Systemic corticosteroid

- Prednisolone 40 mg daily for 5 days followed by 10–20 mg daily for 2 weeks.

- **Erythema Multiforme**

- Doses of prednisolone 0.5–1.0 mg/kg/day tapered over 7–10 days can be given

- **Stevens-Johnson syndrome, Toxic epidermal necrolysis**

- Intermittent administration of high doses of intravenous corticosteroid and cyclophosphamide, (Pulsed therapy)usually three daily doses of dexamethasone (100 mg) or methylprednisolone (500–1000 mg) and a single dose of cyclophosphamide (500 mg) given monthly

ADVERSEEFFECT

a) Side effects of systemic steroids:

- Cushing's habitus
- Osteoporosis
- Growth retardation: in children,
- Hyperglycemia
- May be glycosuria
- Precipitation of diabetes
- Glaucoma

- Posterior Subcapsular cataract may also develop after long term use for several years, especially in children
- Suppression of HPA axis- acute adrenal insufficiency
- Psychiatric disturbances
- Peptic ulceration
- Delayed healing: of wounds and surgical incisions
- Susceptibility to infection, Fragile skin, purple striae, Muscular weakness.[28]

B) <u>Side effects of topical steroids</u>[16,17,28]

I) Local adverse effects of topical steroids

- Thinning of epidermis
- Atrophy
- Telangiectasia, striae
- Easy bruising
- Hypopigmentation,
- Delayed wound healing
- Fungal & bacterial infections
- Candidal infection (25-55%)
- Burning mouth
- Hypogeusia.

Ii)Systemic side effects of topical steroids

- Adrenal pituitary suppression– large amounts applied repeatedly.

CONTRAINDICATIONS: [28]

- Peptic ulcer
- Diabetes mellitus
- Hypertension

- Pregnancy (risk of fetal defects)
- Tuberculosis and other infections
- Osteoporosis
- Herpes simplex keratitis
- Psychosis
- Epilepsy,
- CHF
- Renal failure.

CYCLOSPORINE

Cyclosporine, a cyclic polypeptide consisting of 11 amino acids is produced by the fungus species Beauveria Nivea. It is a Calcineurin Inhibitors.It preferentially inhibits antigen-triggered signal transduction in T lymphocytes, the blunting expression of many lymphokines, including IL-2 and the expression of antiapoptotic proteins. [1,28]

MECHANISM OF ACTION:

Cyclosporine suppresses T-cell-dependent immune mechanisms such as those underlying transplant rejection and some forms of autoimmunity. It preferentially inhibits antigen-triggered signal transduction in T lymphocytes, blunting expression of many lymphokines including IL-2 and the expression of antiapoptotic proteins. Cyclosporine forms a complex with cyclophilin, a cytoplasmic receptor protein present in target cells. This complex binds to calcineurin, inhibiting Ca2+-stimulated dephosphorylation of the cytosolic component of nuclear factor for activated T-cells (NFAT). When cytoplasmic NFAT is dephosphorylated and translocates to the nucleus and complexes with nuclear components required for complete T-cell activation including transactivation of IL-2 and other lymphokine genes. Calcineurin phosphatase activity is inhibited after physical interaction with the cyclosporine/cyclophilin complex. This prevents NFAT dephosphorylation such that NFAT does not enter the nucleus gene transcription is not activated and the T lymphocyte fails to respond to specific antigenic stimulation. Cyclosporine also increases expression of transforming growth factor-b (TGF-b), a potent inhibitor of IL-2-stimulated T-cell proliferation and generation of cytotoxic T lymphocytes (CTL)[1].

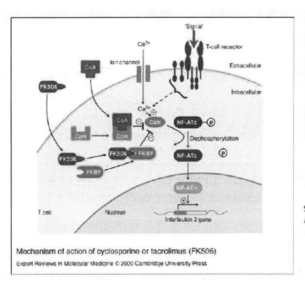

CsA: Cyclosporine

FK506: Tacrolimus

FKBP: FK Binding Protein

CpN: Cyclophilin

NF-AT: Nuclear Factor of Activated T-cells (c- cytosolic component; n- nuclear component).

Stepkowski, *Expert Rev Mol Med*, 2000;2(4):1

Mechanism of action of cyclosporine or tacrolimus (FK506)
Expert Reviews in Molecular Medicine © 2000 Cambridge University Press

PHARMACOKINETICS:

Cyclosporine can be given orally or I.V. Its oral bioavailability is low (about 30%). Food decreases its absorption. It is metabolized by CYP3A which may result in drug-drug interactions. Inactive metabolites are excreted mainly in bile and then in feces but minimally in urine. Plasma half life is about 24 hrs.

INDICATIONS[5]:

- **Recurrent apthous stomatitis /Behcet's syndrome**
- ➢ Topical cyclosporine100mg/ml for moderate cases
- ➢ Systemic cyclosporine 3 to 6 mg/kg/day for chronic case.[34]
- **Lichen planus**
- ➢ Recalcitrant cases of OLP
- ➢ Mouth rinse-5 ml of medication (containing 100 mg of cyclosporine per milliliter) three times daily (i.e., 500-1500mg/day).[35]
- ➢ In a bioadhesive 100 mg/ml, added to the alcohol phase of Zilactin to a final concentration of 0.5 mg/dl. [18,36]

- **Mucous membrane pemphigoid–**
- ➢ 100 mg/ ml can be given.[37]

ADVERSE EFFECTS[1,13,14,28-33]

(Dose-dependent)

- Therapeutic monitoring is essential
- Nephrotoxicity
- (increased by nsaids and aminoglycosides).
- Liver dysfunction.
- Hypertension,
- Hyperkalemia.
- (K-sparing diuretics should not be used).
- Hyperglycemia.
- Viral infections (Herpes - cytomegalovirus).
- Lymphoma (Predispose recipients to cancer).
- Hirsutism
- Neurotoxicity (tremor).

- Gum hyperplasia.
- Anaphylaxis after I.V.
- Headache,
- GI disturbances
- Hypertrichosis.
- Hyperlipidemia
- Hyperuricemia
- Hyper-cholesterolemia
- Diabetogenic
- Elevated LDL cholesterol.

Drug Interactions

O Clearance of cyclosporine is enhanced by co-administration of CYT p 450 inducers *(Phenobarbitone, Phenytoin & Rifampin)*→ rejection of transplant.

O Clearance of cyclosporine is decreased when it is co-administered with *erythromycin or Ketoconazole, Grapefruit juice* → cyclosporine toxicity.

TACROLIMUS (FK506)

Tacrolimus (FK506) is a macrolide antibiotic produced by Streptomyces tsukubaensis. Topical tacrolimus seems to penetrate the skin better than topical cyclosporine[1,28]

It is a fungal macrolide antibiotic.it is Chemically not related to cyclosporine bt both drugs have similar mechanism of action.The internal receptor for tacrolimus is immunophilin (FK-binding protein, FK-BP).

MECHANISM OF ACTION:

Like cyclosporine, tacrolimus inhibits Tcell activation by inhibiting calcineurin. Tacrolimus binds to an intracellular protein FK506-binding protein-12 (FKBP-12) an immunophilin structurally related to cyclophilin. A complex of tacrolimus-FKBP-12, Ca2+, calmodulin, and calcineurin then forms, and calcineurin phosphatase activity is inhibited. As described for cyclosporine the inhibition of phosphatase activity prevents dephosphorylation and nuclear translocation of NFAT and inhibits T-cell activation[1]. (figure as in cyclosporine)

PHARMACOKINETICS:

Tacrolimus can be given orally or I.V. It is 99% metabolized in liver by CYP3A and has a plasma half life of 7-8 hrs.

INDICATIONS:

- **Lichen planus**
  - ➢ 0.1% Tacrolimus application2-4 times a day for 4-8 weeks.
  - ➢ This drug used topically can control symptoms and significantly improve refractory erosive oral LP. [38]
- **Pemphigus Vulgaris/Mucous membrane pemphigoid**
  - ➢ -0.1% tacrolimus ointment twice daily for 3 to 4 week[39]

PHARMACOKINETICS

It is given orally or i.v or topically (ointment).Oral absorption is variable and incomplete, reduced by fat and carbohydrate meals.Half-life after I.V. form is 9-12 hours. It highly bound with serum proteins and concentrated in erythrocytes. It is metabolized by P450 in liver.Excreted mainly in bile and minimally in urine.

ADVERSE EFFECT:[1,13,28,30,40,41]

- Nephrotoxicity(more than csa)

- Neurotoxicity, (tremor, headache, motor disturbances and seizures),(more than csa)

- GI complaints,
- Hypertension,
- Hyperkalemia,
- Hyperglycemia (require insulin).

- Anaphylaxis

Note:

- NO hirsutism or gum hyperplasia
- Drug interactions as cyclosporine.

Differences between csa and TAC?

- TAC is more favorable than csa due to:

- TAC is 10 – 100 times more potent than csa in inhibiting immune responses.

- TAC has decreased episodes of rejection.

- TAC is combined with lower doses of glucocorticoids.

But, TAC is more nephrotoxic and neurotoxic.

SIROLIMUS:

Sirolimus (rapamycin; RAPAMUNE) is a macrocyclic lactone produced by Streptomyces hygroscopicus.

MECHANISM OF ACTION:

Sirolimus inhibits T-lymphocyte activation and proliferation downstream of the IL-2 and other T-cell growth factor receptors. Sirolimus requires formation of a complex with an immunophilin in this case FKBP-12. However, the sirolimus-FKBP-12 complex does not affect calcineurin activity. It binds to and inhibits a protein kinase designated mammalian target of rapamycin (mtor) which is a key enzyme in cell-cycle progression. Inhibition of mtor blocks cell-cycle progression at the G1 to S- phase transition. Pharmacokinetics:

Oral bioavailability is 15%. Fatty meal decreases its bioavailability. Protein binding is 40-45% mainly with albumin. It is extensively metabolized in liver by CYP3A4. Sirolimus is excreted 91% in feces and only 2.5% in urine. Plasma half life is 62 hrs.

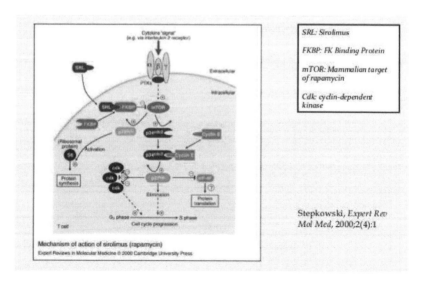

SRL: Sirolimus

FKBP: FK Binding Protein

mTOR: Mammalian target of rapamycin

Cdk: cyclin-dependent kinase

Stepkowski, Expert Rev Mol Med, 2000;2(4):1

Mechanism of action of sirolimus (rapamycin)
Expert Reviews in Molecular Medicine © 2000 Cambridge University Press

INDICATION

Oral lichen planus: There is insufficient evidence to support the use for this indication[42].

ADVERSE EFFECTS:[14,30,44]

- Dose-dependent increase in serum cholesterol and triglycerides,
- Impaired renal function,
- Prolong delayed graft function
- Lymphocele
- Anemia
- Leukopenia.

AZATHIOPRINE:

Azathioprine (IMURAN) is a purine antimetabolite is an immunosuppressive drug. It is an imidazolyl derivative of 6-mercaptopurine. It is used along with a steroid to spare the side effect of long term uses of steroids.Azathioprine is metabolized by thiopurine methyltransferase (TPMT). Ideally the doses should be titrated according to the individual activity of TPMT[1,13,28].

MECHANISM OF ACTION:

Following exposure to nucleophiles such as glutathione, azathioprine is cleaved to 6-mercaptopurine, which in turn is converted to additional metabolites that inhibit de novo purine synthesis. 6-Thio-IMP, a fraudulent nucleotide, is converted to 6-thio-GMP and finally to 6-thio-GTP, which is incorporated into DNA. Cell proliferation is thereby inhibited impairing a variety of lymphocyte functions. [1,28]

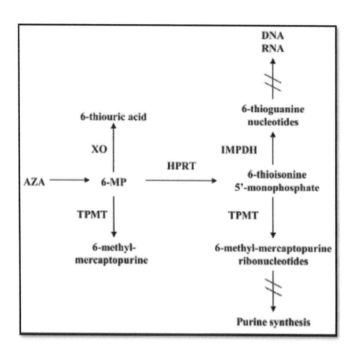

THERAPEUTIC USES:

- **Recurrent aphthous stomatitis /Behcet's syndrome**
- ➤ Used for chronic cases, are non-respondent to primary drugs.
- ➤ 1 to 2 mg/kg/day (100–150 mg/day)[45]
- ➤ Starting with 50 mg/day and escalated up to 150 mg/day. [46]
- **Lichen planus**
- ➤ 50 mg twice daily orally (about 2mg/kg-day) for a period of 3 to 7 months. [47]
- **Pemphigus vulgaris**
- ➤ 0.5–4 mg /kg depending on thiopurine methyltransferase (TPMT) level. [23]
- **Mucous membrane pemphigoid (MMP)**
- ➤ 1–2 mg/kg daily depending on thiopurine methyltransferase levels.[25]

ADVERSE EFFECTS:

- Bone marrow suppression including leukopenia (common)
- Thrombocytopenia (less common)

- And/or anemia (uncommon),
- Increased susceptibility to infections (especially varicella and herpes simplex viruses)
- Hepatotoxicity
- Alopecia
- GI toxicity
- Pancreatitis.

Hence, complete blood count examination before and during azathioprine treatment is mandatory.[1,13,28]

METHOTREXATE

It is an antimetabolite. It suppresses DNA and RNA synthesis during S phase of the cell cycle[28].

MECHANISM OF ACTION

It is a competitive inhibitor of dihydro folate reductase, which is involved in the conversion of folic acid to reduced folate cofactors, required for 1-carbon unit transfers in DNA synthesis. Thus, it inhibits replication and function of T and B lymphocytes. Which in turn prevent the conversion of dihydro folate reductase(DHF) to trihydrofolate (THF). Normally THF is equired in purine and pyramidine synthesis. Thus it suppresses DNA and RNA synthesis. [1,13,28]

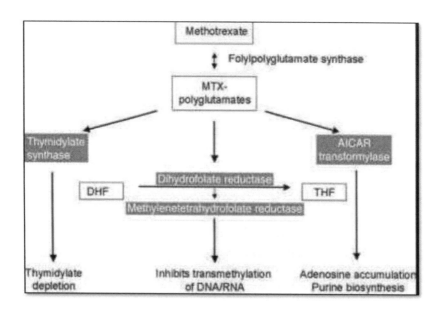

INDICATION:

- **Recurrent aphthous stomatitis /Behcet's syndrome**
  ➢ 7.5 to 20 mg of Methotrexate weekly has been proved to be effective in severe oro-genital lesions. [34]
- **Lichen planus**
  ➢ 7.5-10 mg weekly for 8 weeks. [48]
- **Mucous membrane pemphigoid**
  ➢ The dose ranges from 5 to 25 mg given weekly.
  ➢ Mean duration of the therapy is 15 months, ranging from 8–22 months. [49]

ADVERSE EFFECT: [1,13,28]

- Mylosuppression
- Hepatotoxicity

- Alopecia
- Oral ulceration
- GI disturbances.
- Nausea-vomiting-diarrhea
- Bone marrow depression
- Pulmonary fibrosis
- Renal & hepatic disorders

CYCLOPHOSPHAMIDE

Cyclophosphamide is a unique immunosuppressant as it suppresses B-lymphocyte proliferation but can enhance T-cell responses[1].These drugs are most lethal to rapidly proliferating tissues and appear to cause cell death when they tend to divide. The cytotoxic activity of these drugs correlates with the degree of DNA alkylation.[1,28]

MECHANISM OF ACTION:

Alkylating agents introduce alkyl groups by forming covalent bonds with nucleophilic moieties such as phosphate, sulfhydryl, hydroxyl, carboxyl, amino and imidazole groups present in DNA or RNA. By cross linking in between the strands of DNA they prevent the cell division and protein synthesis. These drugs are most destructive to rapidly proliferating tissues and appear to cause cell death when they tend to divide. The cytotoxicity of these drugs correlates with the degree of DNA alkylation[1].

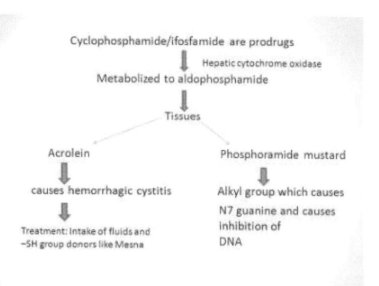

INDICATIONS

- **Pemphigus and mucous membrane pemphigoid-**

➢ Can be used alone i.e.0.5–2 mg/kg daily or with steroid in the form of pulse therapy for severe cases.[49,5]

ADVERSE EFFECTS:[1,13,28,30,51]

- Neutropenia
- Thrombocytopenia
- GIT disorders (Nausea -vomiting-diarrhea)
- Alopecia
- Raised transaminases
- Pancytopenia and hemorrhagic cystitis
- Graftversus-host disease syndrome
- Cardiac toxicity
- Electrolyte disturbances
- Bone marrow suppression
- Sterility (testicular atrophy & amenorrhea)

ETANERCEPT

Etanercept is a complete human Tumor Necrosis Factor-a receptor fusion protein that binds TNF-alpha with greater affinity than the natural receptors. Is genetically engineered fusion protein composed of two soluble tnfp75 receptors moieties linked to Fc portion of human igg1. The drug serves as an exogenously administered soluble TNF-α receptor and provides artificial binding sites to TNF-α. This prevents TNF-α from binding to membrane bound TNFR1 and TNFR2. The drug is used primarily to treat rheumatoid arthritis, and psoriatic arthritis .It is approved for the treatment of inflammatory conditions like ankylosing spondylitis, rheumatoid arthritis, juvenile rheumatoid arthritis, psoriasis arthritis & psoriasis in the USA, Canada, and Europe.[4,53,54]

INDICATION[28,52]

- **For refractory cases of oral lichen planus.**
- Etanercept (2×25 mg/week subcutaneously)
- **Regressed oral ulcer in behçet's disease**.

The rationale for using etanercept in the management of ora lichen planus

The rationale for using etanercept in the management of ora lichen planus is based on the pivotal role of tumor necrosis factor (TNF)-α in the pathogenesis of the disease.[55] Etanercept, a recom binant soluble human TNF receptor protein, competitively inhibits of binding of tnfα to cell surface TNF receptors, thereby preventing TNF-mediated cellular responses.[56] Etanercept is effective in modifying the disease activity of rheumatoid arthritis, juvenilerheumatoid arthritis, psoriasis, and psoriatic arthritis.[56]Use of etanercept for other disorders, such as chronic heart failure, sar-coidosis, ankylosing spondylitis, and Wegener granulomatosis, is also currently being studied.[56] Etanercept is also effective in recurrent aphthous stomatitis[57] and graft-versus-host disease,[58] which share a similar pathogenesis to oral lichen planus. To date, no study has examined the effectiveness of etanercept in the management of oral lichen planus. However, thalidomide, which also inhibits the action of tnfα, is beneficial in the management of generalized lichen planus.[59]

Since etanercept is generally well tolerated, with only a mild-to-moderate reaction at the injection site, this novel therapy seems to be promising. Randomized controlled trials are mandatory to assess the therapeutic value of etanercept in patients with oral lichen planus.

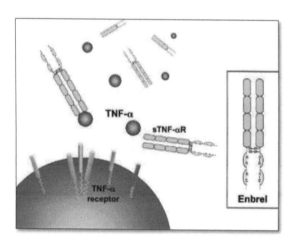

ADVERSE EFFECTS

- Mild to moderate itching,
- Pain,
- Swelling and redness at the site of injection,
- Headache,
- Dizziness,
- Nasal and throat

INFLIXIMAB:

It is a Chimeric monoclonal antibody obtained by exposing the mice to human TNF- α, used to treat autoimmune diseases. The drug cross-links with membrane-bound TNF—α receptors on the cell surface to inhibit T-cell and macrophage function and to prevent the release of other proinflammatory cytokines (IL-1, IL-6 and 8 along with collagenase and metalloproteinases.[28]

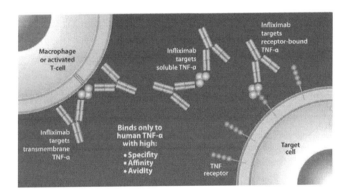

INDICATION

These are advised in cases of refractory and recurrent oral and genital aphthous ulcer in a dose of 5 mg/kg body weight intravenously.[60]

ADVERSE EFFECT[61]

- Leukopenia
- Neutropenia
- Thrombocytopenia
- Pancytopenia (some fatal)

MYCOPHENOLATE MOFETIL:

It is a 2-morpholinoethyl ester of mycophenolic acid[28]

MECHANISM OF ACTION:[1,13,28]

Mycophenolate mofetil is a prodrug that is rapidly hydrolyzed to the active drug, mycophenolic acid (MPA), a selective, noncompetitive and reversible inhibitor of inosine monophosphate dehydrogenase (IMPDH), an important enzyme in the de novo pathway of guanine nucleotide synthesis. B and T lymphocytes are highly dependent on this pathway for cell proliferation while other cell types can use salvage pathways; MPA therefore selectively inhibits lymphocyte proliferation and functions including antibody formation, cellular adhesion, and migration.

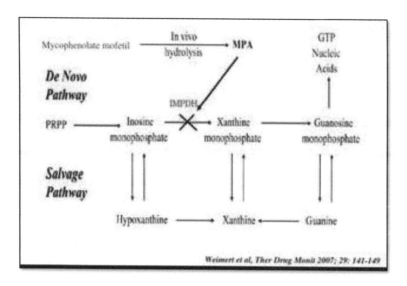

PHARMACOKINETICS:

Mycophenolate mofetil undergoes rapid and complete metabolism to MPA after oral or intravenous administration. MPA, in turn is metabolized to the inactive phenolic glucuronide MPAG. Most (87%) is excreted in the urine as MPA[1].

INDICATION:

- **Lichen planus**
- 2–4 g day33

- **Mucous membrane pemphigoid**
- 35-45 mg/kg/day34
- **Pemphigus Vulgaris-**
- 2-2.5 g/day

ADVERSE EFFECTS: [1,4,1314,28,62,63]

- Leukopenia
- Diarrhea,
- Vomiting, sepsis associated with cytomegalovirus
- Sepsis associated with cytomegalovirus, in combination with mycophenolate mofetil has been associated with devastating viral infections including polyoma nephritis 4,18,28,29.
- GIT toxicity: Nausea, Vomiting, diarrhea, abdominal pain.
- Leukopenia, neutropenia.
- Lymphoma

CONTRAINDICATION

- During pregnancy

BASILIXIMAB

It is a chimeric mouse-human monoclonal antibody to α chain (CD25) of the IL-2receptor of T cells. Basiliximab is an immunosuppressant agent used to prevent immediate transplant rejection in people who are receiving kidney transplants, in combination with other agents. Basiliximab competes with the IL-2 to bind to the alpha chain subunit of the IL2 receptor (CD 25) on the surface of the activated T lymphocytes, hence preventing the receptor from signaling. This prevents T cells from dividing, and also from activating the B cells, that are responsible for the production of antibodies and prevent the expansion of the CD4 and CD8.It is indicated for refractory cases of oral lichen planus[1,28,64]

INDICATION

Oral lichen planus[64]

ADVERSE EFFECT

No short-term side effects have been reported.[65]

EFALIZUMAB

Efalizumab is an antibody (recombinant humanized monoclonal antibody) used as an immunosuppressant in the treatment of psoriasis. It is a monoclonal antibody, binds to the CD11a subunit of lymphocyte functionassociated antigen 1and acts as an immunosuppressant by suppressing lymphocyte activation and the migration of cell out of blood vessels into tissues.[1,28]Efalizumab binds to LFA-1 (lymphocyte function associated antigen) and prevents the LFA-1-ICAM (intercellular adhesion molecule) interaction to block T-cell adhesion, trafficking, and activation.

MECHANISM OF ACTION:

Efalizumab binds to LFA-1 and prevents the LFA-1-ICAM (intercellular adhesion molecule) interaction to block T-cell adhesion, trafficking, and activation[1].

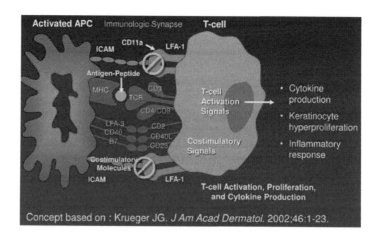

PHARMACOKINETICS[1]:

Pharmacokinetic and pharmacodynamic studies showed that efalizumab produced saturation and 80% modulation of CD11a within 24 hours of therapy

INDICATION[66]

- **Erosive lichen planus**
- An nitial dose of 0.7 mg/kg, followed by a dosage of 1.0 mg/kg per week, approximately 3 weeks had been administered.

ADVERSE EFFECT[28]

- Bacterial sepsis
- Viral meningitis
- Invasive fungal disease.

PIMECROLIMUS

Pimecrolimus is an ascomycin macro lactam derivative. Mechanism of action is similar to tacrolimus i.e. Pimecrolimus attaches to macrophilin-12 (also referred to as FKBP-12) thus inhibiting calcineurin. Pimecrolimus inhibit T-cell activation by stopping the synthesis and release of cytokines from the T-cells. Pimecrolimus also prevent the release of inflammatory cytokines and mediators from mast cells.

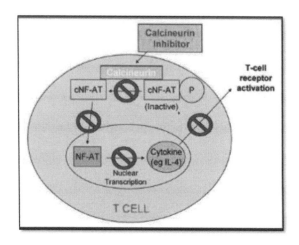

INDICATION[67]

- **Oral lichen planus**
- 1% Pimecrolimus application2-4 times a day for 4-8 weeks has been advised

DIAMINO DIPHENYL SULPHONE (DAPSONE)

Dapsone is a widely used drug in the long-term treatment of leprosy.

INDICATIONS:

- **Recurrent Aphthous stomatitis**
- ➤ Dapsone is given as 100mg orally in divided doses and can be increased at the rate of 50mg/day per week to a maximum dose of 300mg/ day. [68]
- **Mucous membrane pemphigoid**
- ➤ Dapsone 25 mg daily for 3 days, then 50 mg daily for 3 days, then 75 mg per day for 3 days, then 100 mg per day for another 3 days, then rising to 150 mg daily on the seventeenth day.[69]

ADVERSE EFFECT[5]

- ➤ Hemolytic anemia

- ➢ Methemoglobinemia
- ➢ Anemia
- ➢ Agranulocytosis.

MANAGING AND MONITORING PATIENTS TAKING IMMUNOSUPPRESSANTS[86]

Patients need to be under constant surveillance, usually by a partnership between the specialist and the general practitioner. Frequency of visits depends on perceived level of risk, but typical parameters to monitor are summarised in Table 3. Patients may need prophylaxis against the adverse effects of their treatment (Table 4). Therapeutic drug monitoring is available now for a number of drugs, for example cyclosporin, tacrolimus, sirolimus and mycophenolate. This allows for 'concentration-controlled' regimens. Some common drugs, for example corticosteroids, still have no good measure of individual bioavailability.

A. Infection risk Immunosuppression increases susceptibility to infections which can become life-threatening in a matter of hours. At first, common bacterial infections of wounds, chest or urine predominate, but after 1–2 months of therapy opportunistic infections emerge, particularly herpes viruses, pneumocystis pneumonia, fungi and atypical mycobacteria. Vaccinations against influenza (injected) and pneumococcus are recommended in chronically immunosuppressed patients.12 They are safe and reasonably effective when given in the stable maintenance phase. In general, live attenuated virus vaccines, such as varicella or measles, should not be given to immunosuppressed patients (or to close family contacts).

B. Cancer risk In patients taking immunosuppressants, early cancers are often viral induced. They include lymphoproliferative disorders and cervical cancer. In the long term, nearly all common cancers are increased, but particularly skin cancers.

After 20 years of immunoprophylaxis following renal transplant, 80% of Australian patients will have developed skin cancer.

C. Precautions

Seeing a physician regularly while taking immunosuppressant drugs is important. These regular check-ups will allow the physician to make sure the drug is working as it should and to watch for unwanted side effects. These drugs are very powerful and can cause serious side effects, such as high blood pressure, kidney problems and liver problems. Some side effects may not show up until years after the medicine is used. Anyone who has been advised to take immunosuppressant drugs should thoroughly discuss the risks and benefits with the prescribing physician.

Immunosuppressant drugs lower a person's resistance to infection and can make infections harder to treat. The drugs can also increase the chance of uncontrolled bleeding. Anyone who has a serious infection or injury while taking immunosuppressant drugs should get prompt medical attention and should make sure that the treating physician knows about the immunosuppressant prescription. The prescribing physician should be immediately informed if signs of infection, such as fever or chills, cough or hoarseness, pain in the lower back or side, or painful or difficult urination, bruising or bleeding, blood in the urine, bloody or black, tarry stools occur. Other ways of preventing infection and injury include washing the hands frequently, avoiding sports in which injuries may occur, and being careful when using knives, razors, fingernail clippers or other sharp objects. Avoiding contact with people who have infections is also important. In addition, people who are taking or have been taking immunosuppressant drugs should not have immunizations, such as smallpox vaccinations, without checking with their physicians. Because of their low resistance to infection, people taking these drugs might get the disease that the vaccine is designed to prevent. People taking immunosuppressant drugs also should avoid contact with anyone who has taken the oral polio vaccine, as there is a chance the virus could be passed on to them. Other people living in their home should not take the oral polio vaccine.

Immunosuppressant drugs may cause the gums to become tender and swollen or to bleed. If this happens, a physician or dentist should be notified. Regular brushing, flossing, cleaning and gum massage may help prevent this problem. A dentist can provide advice on how to clean the teeth and mouth without causing injury.

D. Special conditions People who have certain medical conditions or who are taking certain other medicines may have problems if they take immunosuppressant drugs. Before taking these drugs, the prescribing physician should be informed about any of these conditions:

E. Allergies Anyone who has had unusual reactions to immunosuppressant drugs in the past should let his or her physician know before taking the drugs again. The physician should also be told about any allergies to foods, dyes, preservatives, or other substances.

F. Pregnancy Azathioprine may cause birth defects if used during pregnancy, or if either the male or female is using it at time of conception. Anyone taking this medicine should use a barrier method of birth control, such as a diaphragm or condoms. Birth control pills should not be used without a physician's approval. Women who become pregnant while taking this medicine should check with their physicians immediately. The medicine's effects have not been studied in humans during pregnancy. Women who are pregnant or who may become pregnant and who need to take this medicine should check with their physicians.

G. Breastfeeding Immunosuppressant drugs pass into breast milk and may cause problems in nursing babies whose mothers take it. Breastfeeding is not recommended for women taking this medicine.

H. Other Medical Conditions

People who have certain medical conditions may have problems if they take immunosuppressant drugs. For example: People who have shingles (herpes zoster) or chickenpox, or who have recently been exposed to chickenpox, may develop severe disease in other parts of their bodies when they take these medicines; The medicine's effects may be greater in people with kidney disease or liver disease, because their bodies are slow to get rid of the medicine. The effects of oral forms of this medicine may be weakened in people with intestinal problems, because the medicine cannot be absorbed into the body. Before using immunosuppressant drugs, people with these or other medical problems should make sure their physicians are aware of their conditions.

I. Use of Certain Medicines Taking immunosuppressant drugs with certain other drugs may affect the way the drugs work or may increase the chance of side effects.

J. Side effects Increased risk of infection is a common side effect of all the immunosuppressant drugs. The immune system protects the body from infections and when the immune system is suppressed, infections are more likely. Taking such antibiotics as co-trimoxazole prevents some of these infections. Immunosuppressant drugs are also associated with a slightly increased risk of cancer because the immune system also plays a role in protecting the body against some forms of cancer. For example, long-term use of immunosuppressant drugs carries an increased risk of developing skin cancer as a result of the combination of the drugs and exposure to sunlight.

Other side effects of immunosuppressant drugs are minor and usually go away as the body adjusts to the medicine. These include loss of appetite, nausea or vomiting, increased hair growth, and trembling or shaking of the hands. Medical attention is not necessary unless these side effects continue or cause problems.

K. Interactions Immunosuppressant drugs may interact with other medicines. When this happens, the effects of one or both drugs may change or the risk of side effects may be greater. Other drugs may also have an adverse effect on immunosuppressant therapy. This is particularly important for patients taking cyclosporin or tacrolimus. For example, some drugs can cause the blood levels to rise, while others can cause the blood levels to fall and it is important to avoid such contraindicated combinations. Other examples are:

- The effects of azathioprine may be greater in people who take allopurinol, a medicine used to treat gout.
- A number of drugs, including female hormones (estrogens), male hormones (androgens), the antifungal drug ketoconazole (Nizoral), the ulcer drug cimetidine (Tagamet) and the erythromycins (used to treat infections), may increase the effects of cyclosporine.
- When sirolimus is taken at the same time as cyclosporin, the blood levels of sirolimus may be increased to a level where there are severe side effects. Although these two drugs are usually used together, the sirolimus should be taken four hours after the dose of cyclosporin.
- Tacrolimus is eliminated through the kidneys. When the drug is used with other drugs that may harm the kidneys, such as cyclosporin, the antibiotics gentamicin and amikacin, or the antifungal drug amphotericin B, blood levels of tacrolimus may be increased. Careful kidney monitoring is essential when tacrolimus is given with any drug that might cause kidney damage.
- The risk of cancer or infection may be greater when immunosuppressant drugs are combined with certain other drugs which also lower the body's ability to fight disease and infection. These drugs include corticosteroids such as prednisone; the anticancer drugs chlorambucil (Leukeran), cyclophosphamide (Cytoxan) and mercaptopurine (Purinethol); and the monoclonal antibody muromonab-CD3 (Orthoclone), which also is used to prevent transplanted organ rejection.

IMMUNOSTIMULANTS

CLASSIFICATION OF IMMUNOSTIMULANT

According to Patil US et al 2012[1]

I.   Bacillus Calmette-Guerin (BCG):

II.   Levamisole

III. Thalidomide

IV.   Recombinant Cytokines

- Interferons
- Interleukins
- Colony stimulating factors

According to Pagare SS et al[13]

I.   Immunostimulants Increasing the humoral antibody responses

- Amantadine
- Tilorone BCG vaccine

II.   Enhancing the phagocytic activity of macrophages

- Recombinant cytokines

-interferons

- interleukin-2

III. Modifying the cell mediated immune responses

- Thalidomide
- Levamisole

IMMUNOSTIMULANTS

THALIDOMIDE

Thalidomide was first marketed in West Germany in the year 1957 with the trade-name Contergan. A German drug company named Chemie Grunenthal developed and prescribed as a sedative or hypnotic and antiemetic for the treatment of morning sickness. But now due to its immunomodulatory action it is used for a number of conditions including: multiple myeloma, erythema nodosum leprosum and a number of other cancers, Crohn's disease, sarcoidosis, graft-versus-host disease, rheumatoid arthritis, & for some symptoms of HIV/AIDS. [1,28]

MECHANISM OF ACTION:

It inhibits TNF-α, IL-6, IL10 and IL-12 production, modulates the production of IFN-γ and increases the production of IL-2, IL4 and IL-5 by the cells of immune system. It increases lymphocyte count, costimulates T cells and modulates natural killer cell cytotoxicity. It also inhibits NF-κband COX-2 activity.[1,28]

INDICATIONS:

- **Recurrent Aphthous stomatitis**
➢   100 to 200 mg/day to start with and to be continued till remission, followed by a maintenance dose of 50 to 100 mg daily or 50 mg every other day.[70]
- **Lichen planus**
➢   It is an effective treatment of severe corticosteroid resistant erosive oral lichen planus cases.
➢   Topical- Thalidomide 1% paste (150 mg Thalidomide powder dissolved in pure glycerol into a paste)Apply 3 times/day for 1 week

> Systemic-Initial dose of 50 to 100 mg/day. [71]

CONTRAINDICATIONS:[1,28]

- Known hypersensitivity to thalidomide,
- Pregnancy or breastfeeding
- Patient age < 12 years, Patients who are unable or unwilling to comply with required contraceptive measures.

ADVERSE EFFECT:[1,28]

- Teratogenicity causes phycomelia (due to antiangigenesis and inactivation of the protein cereblon)
- Somnolence
- Edema
- Hypotension,
- Headache,
- Haematuria
- Arthralgia
- Myalgia,
- Increased bilirubin
- Neutropenia
- Leucopenia
- Lymphopenia
- Constipation
- Peripheral neuropathy
- Dizziness
- Paraesthesia

Patient should undergo STEPS (System for Thalidomide Education and Prescribing Safety) before prescribing this drug.

LEVAMISOLE

Levamisole (ERGAMISOL) a heterocyclic compound was synthesized originally as an anthelmintic, but appears to restoredepressed immune function of B lymphocytes, T lymphocytes, monocytes and macrophages[28,72].

MECHANISM OF ACTION[1,13,28]

Physiologically, thymopoietin affects many components of the immune system including both neutrophils, macrophages and lymphocytes and its therapeutically important actions are probably targeted at stimulation of phagocytosis and stimulation of regulatory T cells to restore homeostasis in a disturbed immune system. Levamisole mimic the thymic hormone thymopoetin, so form thymopoietin – mimetic tertiary structure which stimulate lymphocyte by its iidazole component. It also potentiates the activity of human interferon, inhibit aerobic tumour glycolysis.

INDICATION

- **Aphthous**
- ➢ 150mg/day with or without combination with steroids (15 mg Prednisolone). [73]
- **Lichenplanus**
- ➢ 150- 300 mg/day for 3 months (Monotherapy) [74]
- ➢ 150 mg/day levamisole and 15 mg/day Prednisolone for 3 consecutive days each week. [75]
- Mucous membrane pemphigoid
- ➢ Dose ranging from 5 to 25 mg given weekly.
- ➢ Mean duration of the therapy is15 months, ranging from 8–22 months.[49]

ADVERSE EFFECTS: [1,4,13,28]

- Flu-like symptoms
- Allergic manifestation
- Nausea

- Muscle pain
- GI disturbances
- Headache
- Dizziness
- Insomnia
- Thrombocytopenia
- Granulocytopenia

BACILLUS CALMETTE-GUERIN (BCG)

Live bacillus Calmette-Guerin (BCG) is an attenuated, live culture of the bacillus of Calmette and Guerin strain of Mycobacterium bovis. The cytotoxic effect of BCG could result from the direct action of the CD4 cells or from the cytotoxic effect of the released cytokines and the activation of other cytotoxic cells [cytolytic Tlymphocytes, macrophages, natural killer or lymphokineactivated killer cells].[1,28]

MECHANISM OF ACTION:

Induction of a granulomatous reaction at the site of administration.

INDICATION[76]

- Erosive lichen planus
- ➢ Intralesional injection of 0.5 ml BCG-PSN every other day for 2 weeks can be administered

ADVERSE EFFECTS [4,30]

- Hypersensitivity
- Shock
- Chills
- Fever
- Malaise
- Immune complex disease.

INTERFERON

Interferons are compounds produced by the body that perform functions related to the immune system, which is the body's defense against invading pathogens. Recombinant interferon refers to interferon compounds produced by the recombinant techniques. Interferon causes induction of certain enzymes by binding to cell surface receptors, inhibition of cell proliferation, and enhancement of immune activities, including increased phagocytosis by macrophages and augmentation of specific cytotoxicity by T lymphocytes[1,28].

MECHANISM OF ACTION

Induction of certain enzymes, inhibition of cell proliferation, and enhancement of immune activities, including increased phagocytosis by macrophages and augmentation of specific cytotoxicity by T lymphocytes[1]

INDICATION

- **For Behcet's syndrome[77]**

➤ Intermediate (e.g. 6×10^6 IU thrice a week) or high doses (e.g. 9×10^6 IU thrice a week) of Interferon alpha 2 a (Roferon A) and b (Intron A) are principally more effective than low doses (3×10^6 IU thrice a week)

➤ Lower doses are recommended as a maintenance therapy when treatment is successful in the first 1 to 4 month

Oral submucous fibrosis[78].

➤ Intralesional injection of interferon gamma (0.01– 10.0 U/ml) 3 times a day for 6 months can be given.

ADVERSE EFFECTS[1]

➤ Hypotension

➤ Arrhythmias

➤ Rarely cardiomyopathy and myocardial infarction

➤ GI distress

➤ Anorexia

➤ Weight loss

- ➤ Myalgia
- ➤ Depression.

COLCHICINE

Colchicine suppresses the cell-mediated immune responses.

MECHANISM OF ACTION

Inhibits cell-mediated immune responses, by inhibiting Ig secretion, IL-1 production, histamine release and HLA-DR expression

PHARMACOKINETICS

Rapidly absorbed when taken orally; peak plasma levels are reached 30 - 120 min after ingestion. • 50% of the drug circulates and links to plasma proteins. • Metabolized in the liver, and the majority is eliminated through bile in the feces. • Also distributed in spleen and kidney. • Overall, 10-20% of the dose is eliminated unchanged in the urine.

INDICATION

- **Aphthous ulcers**[79]

➤ In a more recent open study of 20 patients, colchicine (1.5 mg/day for 2 months) produced a significant decrease in the pain scores and frequency of the self-reported aphthous ulcers.

➤ Unfortunately, not all the patients get benefit from the colchicine therapy, and at least 20% have the painful gastrointestinal symptoms or diarrhea, and can affect the reproductive system (causing infertility) in young males.

➤ Combined colchicine and thalidomide therapy may provide an occasional benefit in the recalcitrant RAS.

HERBAL MEDICINAL PLANTS AS AN IMMUNOMODULATOR

Indian and worldwide medicinal studies have reported a large number of plants included to promote the physical mental and defense mechanism in the body. On other hand a large number of medicinal plants included in Rasayanas have been claimed to possess immunomodulatory activities. Medicinal plants which are used as immunomodulatory effect to provide alternative potential to conventional hemotherapy for a variety of diseases, especially in relation to host defense mechanism. The use of plant product like polysaccharides, lectins, peptides, flavonoids and tannins has been the immune response or immune system in various in-vitro and in-vivo models. The immune system is a part of body which detects the pathogen by using a specific receptor to produce immediately response by the activation of immune components cells, cytokines, chemokines and also release of inflammatory mediator. In the innate immune the nature killer cell plays an important role to the defiance against virus-infected and malignant cell to destroy the abnormal cells. The drug affecting the immune system is termed as immunomodulatory or adaptigenic. Some repress the system and are value in, for example, preventing rejection of transplanted organs and other are stimulating and can be used to help combat viral infection such as AIDS or assist in the treatment of cancer. Also, the use of natural immunomodulators in synergy with existing drugs may involve the functional manipulation of multiple molecular targets leading to improved therapeutic efficacy and reduced toxicity[80].Plant extracts used in traditional therapy are being reviewed for their chemo protective and Immunomodulatory activities. Immunomodulators are biological response modifiers; exert their antitumor effects by improving host defense mechanisms against the tumor. They have a direct anti-proliferative effect on tumour cells and also enhance the ability of the host to tolerate damage by toxic chemicals that may be used to destroy cancer.[81]

Immunomodulatory therapy could provide an alternative to conventional chemotherapy for a variety of diseased conditions, especially when host's defense mechanisms have to be activated under the conditions of impaired immune responsiveness or when a selective immunosuppression has to be induced in a situation.

MECHANISM OF ACTION OF THE RASAYANAS/ IMMUNOMODULATORS

It has been reported that the "Rasayanas" are rejuvena- tors, nutritional supplements and possess strong antioxi- dant activities. They also exert antagonistic action on oxidative stressors, giving rise to the formation of different free radicals. They are used mainly to combat the effects of ageing, atherosclerosis, cancer, diabetes, rheumatoid arthritis, autoimmune disease and Parkinson's disease. The Rasayana herbs seem to operate through immunostimulant, immunoadjuvant, and immunosuppressant activities or by affecting the effector arm of the immune response.[82] Mechanisms of immunomodulation activity occur mainly via phagocytosis stimulation, macrophages activation, immunostimulatory effect on peritoneal macrophages, lymphoid cells stimulation, cellular immune function enhancement and nonspecific cellular immune system effect, antigen-specific immunoglobulin production increase, increased nonspecific immunity mediators and natural killer cell numbers, reducing chemotherapy-induced leukopenia, and increasing circulating total white cell counts and interleukin-2 levels[83]

Modulation of the immune responses through the stimulatory or suppressive activity of a phyto-extract may help maintain a disease-free state in normal or unhealthy people. Agents that activate host defense mechanisms in the presence of an impaired immune response can provide supportive therapy to conventional chemotherapy.[84]

Many studies have reported the identification of immunomodulatory compounds with pharmacological activity and a limited toxicity. In this context, ethnopharmacology represents the most important way possible to uncover interesting and therapeutically helpful molecules. The phytochemical analysis of Rasayana plants has revealed a large number of compounds including tannic acid, flavo- noids, tocopherol, curcumin, ascorbate, carotenoids, polyphenols, etc., which have been shown to have potent immunomodulatory properties. The herbal mixture prepa- rations of Indian traditional medicine may stimulate immunomodulation due to their content of plants with immunomodulatory properties that probably act synergistically. This hypothesis along with the lack of toxicity can be important to understand their use in the past as well as currently.[85]

From the review of many studies it should be evident that there are many medicinal plants which exert immunomodulatory activity in experimental models at a particular dose. Different types of screening methods both *in vivo* and *in vitro* have been employed to determine their pharma- cological activity. Some medicinal plants may stimulate the immune system, and some may suppress the immune response. Also, various secondary metabolites exhibit a wide range of immunomodulating activity[83].

Methods for Testing Immunological Factors[81]

The routine process for screening is to extract single ingredient or single distilled fraction from herbal drugs, determine its bioactivity by the classic pharmacological means. The whole animal model is the most classic pharmacological screening model, which is very important at the aspect of medicine evaluation because it can apparently respond to the efficacy, side effect and toxicity of medicines in whole. Although this method is high cost and low efficient, at present it is still a primary way to drug discovery and evaluation.

Several in vitro, in vivo methods of pharmacological screening of medicinal plants having immunomodulatory activity have been done.

In vitro methods:

1. Inhibition of histamine release from mast cells

2. Mitogens induced lymphocyte proliferation

3. Inhibition of T cell proliferation

4. Chemiluminescence in macrophages

5. PFC (plaque forming colony) test in vitro

6. Inhibition of dihydro-orotate dehydrogenase

In vivo methods:

1. Spontaneous autoimmune diseases in animals

2. Acute systemic anaphylaxis in rats

3. Anti-anaphylactic activity (Schultz-Dale reaction)

4. Passive cutaneous anaphylaxis

5. Arthus type immediate hypersensitivity

6. Delayed type hypersensitivity

7. Reversed passive arthus reaction

8. Adjuvant arthritis in rats

9. Collagen type II induced arthritis in rats

10. Proteoglycan-induced progressive polyarthritis in mice

11. Experimental autoimmune thyroiditis

12. Coxsackievirus B3-induced myocarditis

13. Porcine cardiac myosin-induced autoimmune myocarditis in rats

14. Experimental allergic encephalomyelitis

15. Acute graft versus host disease (GVHD) in rats

16. Influence on SLE-like disorder in MRL/lpr mice

17. Prevention of experimentally induced myasthenia gravis in rats

18. Glomerulonephritis induced by antibasement membrane antibody in rats

19. Auto-immune uveitis in rats

20. Inhibition of allogenic transplant rejection.

CURCUMA LONGA:

Biological source: Turmeric consists of dried as well as fresh rhizomes of the plant known as Curcuma longa belonging to family zingeiberaceae. It contains not less than 1.5 % of curcumin. It acts as immunostimulant.

Geographical source: curcuma is a genous of about 70 species of rhizomatous herbs distributed in South East Asia and especially India, China, Italy, Malaysia, Australia. In India, it accounts for as much as 90 % of total output of the world.

Tamil Nadu and Andhra Pradesh together contribute about 70 % of the Indian production [87].

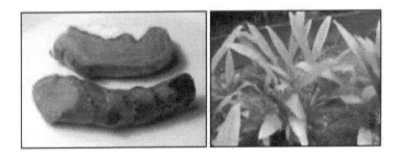

Chemical constituents: Turmeric contains about 5 % volatile oil, resin and yellow coloring substances known as curcuminoids. The chief component of curcuminoids is known as curcumin (50-60 %) structure is mentioned in Fig. And some sesquiterpenes such as α and β pinene, zingiberene.

FIG. 3: CURCUMIN

Chemical test: The aqueous solution of turmeric with boric acid gives reddish brown color on addition of alkali changes to greenish blue. With acetic anhydride and conc. Sulphuric acid gives violet color.

INDICATIONS

o **Oral Sub-mucous fibrosis**[88]

o **Gingivitis**[95]

CONTRA-INDICATIONS:

Hypersensitivity to any of the ingredients. The safety in Pregnancy & Lactation has not been established

DRUGINTERACTIONS

No clinically relevant interactions have been reported so far.

ALOE VERA:

Biological source: Aloes is the dried juice of the leaves of Aloe barbadensis, Aloe perryi, Aloe ferox, aloe Africana and Aloe spicata belonging to family liliaceae. Geographical source: Aloe is endogenous to eastern and southern Africa and grown in cape colony, Zanzibar and island of Socotra. It is also cultivated in Caribbean island, Europe and many parts of India [14,83].

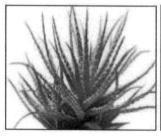 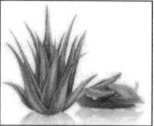

Chemical constituents: All the varieties of aloe are the major source of anthraquinone glycosides. The principal active composition of aloe is aloin, which is a mixture of glycoside among barbaloin is the chief constituent (structure is mentioned in Fig.). The drug also contains aloetic acid, homonataloin, aloesone, chrysamminic acid etc[90,91].

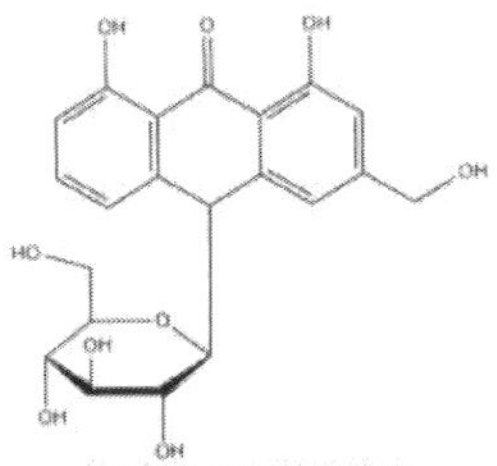

FIG. 10: BARBALOIN

Chemical test: The chemical tests for aloes are performed either for general detection or detection of specific variety of aloes.

General test: For these tests, 1 g of aloe powder is boiled with 10 ml water and filtered with help of kieselguhr. The filtrate is used for bromine test and Schoenteten's reaction.

Bromine test: Freshly prepared bromine solution is added to a small quantity of above filtrate. The test gives a pale yellow precipitate to tetrabromalin.

Borax test: Little quantity of above filtrate is treated with borax and shaken well till the borax dissolves. When few drops of this solution added to a test tube nearly filled with water a green fluorescence appears.

Special test: These tests are meant for distinguishing varieties of aloe vera.

Nitrous acid test: Crystal of sodium nitrate along with small quantity of acetic acid is added to aqueous solution of aloes.

Curacao aloe – sharp pink to carmine color

Cape aloe – faint pink color

Zanzibar aloe – very less change in color

Nitric acid test: This test carried out either by directly applying nitric acid to drug or to its aqueous solution.

Curacao aloes – deep brownish red color

Cape aloes – brownish color changing to green

Socotrine aloe – pale brownish to yellow color

Zanzibar aloes – yellowish brown color

Modified anthraquinone test: The aqueous solution of aloes is treated with ferric chloride solution and dilute hydrochloric acid to bring out the oxidative hydrolysis of aloe emodine. The hydrolysis sets free anthraquinones which are collected in organic solvent like carbon tetrachloride.The organic layer is separated and shaken with dilute ammonia. The ammonical layer rose – pink to cherry red color.

INDICATION

Radiation induced mucositis and candidiasis.[92]

SIDE EFFECTS

Topical

It may cause redness, burning and stinging sensation. Allergic reactions are mostly due to anthraquinones, such as aloin and barbaloin. It is best to apply in a small area first to test for possible allergic reaction.[93]

Systemic

Abdominal cramps, diarrhea, red urine, hepatitis, dependency or worsening of constipation. Prolonged use has been reported to increase the risk of colorectal cancer. Laxative effect may cause electrolyte imbalances (low potassium levels).[92]

OCIMUM SANCTUM:

Biological source: Tulsi consist of fresh and dried leaves of Ocimum sanctum belonging to family lamiaceae. It contains not less than 0.40 % eugenol.

The fresh leaves are used as stimulant, aromatic, anticatarrhal, spasmolytic, skin disease. The drug is a good immunomodulatory agent [1]

Geographical source: It is an herbaceous, much branched annual plant found throughout India. It is considered as sacred by Hindu's. The plant is commonly cultivated in garden and also grown near temples. It is propagated by seed [96]

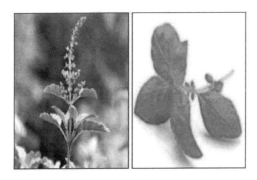

Chemical constituents: Tulsi leaves contains pleasant volatile oil (0.1 – 0.9%). It contains approximately 70 % eugenol, carvacrol (3%) (fig. 9) and caryophyllin also present.

FIG. 9: EUGENOL   CARVACROL

INDICATION

- **Lichen planus**[97]

SIDE EFFECTS

- Uterine contraction during pregnancy [98]
- May add to the effect of diabetic medication [99]
- May stain teeth [100]

SPIRULINA

Biological and geographical source: Spirulina, a blue-green algae (cyanophytes/cyanobacteria), grows as microscopic, corkscrew-shaped multicellular filaments and is now classified as a distinct genus, Arthrospira. A. Platensis is found in Africa and Asia, and A. Maxima is found in Central America.[101,102] Free growing, spirulina exists only in high-salt alkaline water in subtropical and tropical areas, sometimes imparting a dark-green color to bodies of water.[103] Spirulina is noted for its characteristic behavior in carbonated water and energetic growth in laboratory cultures.[104] It is commercially grown in the United States and has been proposed as a primary foodstuff to be cultivated during long-term space missions because it withstands extreme conditions.[105]Due to its unique growth requirements, contamination of open pond cultures of spirulina by other microorganisms is usually slight, with the alga growing as a relatively pure culture.

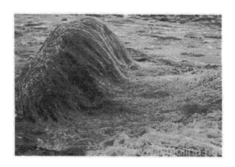

INDICATION[106]

- Osmf

- Lukoplakia

ADVERSE EFFECT

Few reports of adverse reactions are available. Case reports of immunoblistering[107] and rhabdomyolysis[108] linked to spirulina have been published. Cyanobacteria (blue-green algae) may contain the amino acid phenylalanine; therefore, people with phenylketonuria should avoid spirulina. A case of spirulina-associated hepatotoxicity has been reported.[108] Hepatotoxic microcystins and neurotoxic anatoxin-a are produced by a number of cyanobacteria and have been reported as spirulina contaminants.[109,110] Other contaminants include the heavy metals mercury, cadmium, arsenic, and lead, as well as microbes cultivated on fermented animal waste.[111] There may be a potential for adverse reactions in people with autoimmune disorders who consume immunostimulatory herbal preparations.[112]

CONCLUSION

Immunology is probably one of the most rapidly developing areas of medical research and has great promises with regard to the prevention and treatment of a wide range of disorders of the oral cavity. Immunomodulators are going to be a core part of the next generation clinical medicine. Helping the body help itself by optimizing the immune system is of central importance in a society so stressed, unhealthily nourished and exposed to toxins that most of us are likely to have compromised immune systems. Immunomodulating agents are natural or synthetic substances, which by altering the immune system affect therapeutic benefits. They are introduced into the body which activates macrophages and granulocytes, there by increasing phagocytosis. Immunomodulating drugs play a major role not only in Allopathic drug system as well in Homeopathic systems. Many immunomodulating drugs are available in the market. It is envisaged that these products will in first instance primarily comprise product for long term treatment such as treatment of HIV, tumor &organ transplantation also in specific immunotherapy. As Natural drugs are specific in only enhance phagocytosis & lymphocyte proliferation. In compare to that Synthetic & Semisynthetic drugs are non specific; acts by inhibitition of DNA synthesis and regulating both B & T cell lymphocytes. However it is required to develop such new synthetic drugs which are devoid of hypersensitivity and other allergic response. More newer Immunomodulating agents should develop which are helpful in treating autoimmune diseases without any side effects.

The use of various plant extracts and herbal fed additives in specific dose during the scheduled vaccination regimen may be helpful in obtaining higher protective antibody against different infections including production and development of more effective cell mediate immune response for protection against various bacterial, viral and other diseases. Herbal formulation may be therefore recommended for use as positive immunomodulator. There are several botanical products with potential therapeutic applications because of their high efficacy, low cost and low toxicity.Immunomodulation using medicinal plants could supply alternate predictable chemotherapy for different diseases, particularly once there is a weakened immune response and when discriminatory immunosuppression happens, as in the case of autoimmune syndromes. There is intense activity to detect additional particular immunomodulators that imitate or antagonize the biological properties of interleukins and cytokines. Improvement of evaluation of these mediators will create sensitive and specific screenss. We should reconsider natural medications that could be important sources of innovative ligands capable of directing specific cellular receptors.

REFERENCES

1.   Patil US, Jaydeokar AV, Bandawane DD. Immunomodulators: A Pharmacological Review. Int J Pharm Pharm Sci, 2012 Vol 4, Suppl 1, 30-36.

2.   Patchen ML, D'Alesandro MM, Glucan IB. Mechanisms involved in its radioprotective effect. J. Leuk. Biol. 1987; 42: 95-105.

3.   Benny KH, Vanitha J. Immunomodulatory and Antimicrobial Effects of Some Traditional Chinese Medicinal Herbs: A Review. Current Medicinal Chemistry. 2004; 11: 1423-1430.

4.   Sharma HL, Sharma K.K. Principals of Pharmacology. 1st ed. Paras Medical Publishers, New Delhi; 2007: 428-453.

5.   Shivhare P, Shankarnarayan L, Singh A, Patil ST, Yadav M. Role of Immunomodulators in Oral Diseases. Int J Oral Health Med Res 2015;2(3):73-80.

6.   Alamgir M, Uddin SJ. Recent advances on the ethnomedicinal plants as immunomodulatory agents. Ethnomedicine: A Source of Complementary Therapeutics. 2010; 227-244.

7.   Arokiyaraj S, Perinbam K. Immunosuppressive effect of kolli hills on mitogen-stimulated proliferation of the human peripheral blood mononuclear cells in vitro. Indian J Pharmacol. 2007; 39: 180-183.

8.   Salem ML. Immunomodulatory and therapeutic properties of the Nigella sativa L. seed. International Immunopharmacology 2005; 5: 1749-1770.

9.   Quinn MT, Scheptkin IA, Wiley JA, Macrophage immunomodulatory activity of polysaccharides isolated from Juniperus scopolorum. International Immunopharmacology 2005; 5: 1783-1799.

10.   Zang Y, Ting Li and Jia W. Distinct immunosuppressive effect by Isodon serra extracts. International Immunopharmacology 2005; 5: 1957-1965.

11.   Malfitano AM, Matarese G, Pisanti S. Arvanil inhibits T lymphocyte activation and ameliorates autoimmune encephalomyelitis. J Neuroimmunol. 2006; 171: 1-2.

12.   Shrivastava et al. herbal immunomodulors: a review, IJPSR, 2014; Vol. 5(4): 1192-1207.

13.   Pagare SS, SinghiR, Vahanwala S, Nayak CD. Rationale in usage of immunomodulators for management of head, face and neck cancers. International Journal of Head and Neck Surgery, September-December 2012; 3(3):154-157.

14.   Katzung G. Bertram: Basic and Clinical Pharmacology. 10th edition: Mc. graw-Hill companies; year: 2011; 87-85.

15.   Kokate C.K., Purohit A.P., Gokhale S.B: Text book of Pharmacognosy. 45th edition Nirali Prakashan; 2012: 8.4- 8.56, 7.35.

16.   Kallali B et al. Corticosteroids in dentistry. Indian acad ora med 2011;23(2):128-131.

17.   Vijayavel T et al. Corticosteroids in oral diseases. Indian Journal of Drugs and Diseases. 2012;1(7):168-170.

18.   Lodi G, Scully C,Carrozzo M, Griffiths M,. Sugerman PB, Thongprasom K.Current controversies in oral lichen planus: Report of an international consensus meeting. Part 2. Clinical management and malignant transformation.Oral Surg Oral Med Oral Pathol Oral Radiol Endod 2005;100:164-78.

19.   Randell S, Cohen L. Erosive lichen planus. Management of oral lesions with intralesional corticosteroid injections. J Oral Med 1974;29:88-91.

20.   Carbone M, Goss E, Carrozzo M, Castellano S, Conrotto D, Broccoletti R, et al. Systemic and topical corticosteroid treatment of oral lichen planus: a comparative study with longterm follow-up. J Oral Pathol Med 2003;32:323-9.

21.   Rajendran R et al. Cell-mediated and humoral immune responses in oral submucous fibrosis (OSMF). Cancer, 1986, 58: 2628-263.

22.   Scully C, Gorsky M, Lozada-Nur FL.The diagnosis and management of recurrent aphthous stomatitis A consensus approach J Am Dent Assoc 2003;134(2):200-207.

23.   Harman KE, Alberts Black MM, et al. Guidelines for the management of pemphigus vulgaris. British Journal of Dermatology 2003; 149: 926–937.

24. Ratnam KV, Phay KL, Tan CK. Pemphigus therapy with oral prednisolone regimens. Int J Dermatol 1990; 29: 363–7.

25. ScullyC, Muzio LL. Oral mucosal diseases: Mucous membrane pemphigoid. British Journal of Oral and Maxillofacial Surgery 46 (2008) 358–366.

26. Crispian Scully, Jose Baganb. Oral mucosal diseases: Erythema multiforme. British Journal of Oral and Maxillofacial Surgery2008;46: 90–5.

27. Kardaun SH, Jonkman MF.Dexamethasone Pulse Therapy for Stevens-Johnson Syndrome/Toxic Epidermal Necrolysis. Acta Derm Venereol 2007; 87: 144–148.

28. Brunton LL, Parker KL, Blumenthal DK, Buxton ILO.Goodman & Gilman's Manual of Pharmacology and Therapeutics.McGraw-Hill.2008.

29. Sharma HL, Sharma K.K. Principals of Pharmacology. 1st ed. Paras Medical Publishers, New Delhi; 2007: 428-453.

30. Goodman & Gilman's. Manual of Pharmacology and Therapeutics, Professor of Pharmacology & Medicine University of California, 5th ed. San Diego LaJolla, California 2008; 262-279.

31. Jain S. Handbook of Pharmacology. 3rd ed. Pars Publication. 2008; 595-609.

32. Tortora GJ and Derrickson BP. Principles of Anatomy and Physiology. Vol-1. 12th ed. 2008; 846-852.

33. Chaudhuri SK. Quintessence of Medical Pharmacology .2nd ed. 2001; 103-106.

34. Altenburg A, Abdel-Naser MB, Seeber H, Abdallah M, Zouboulis CC.Practical aspects of management of recurrent aphthous stomatitis. J Eur Acad Dermatol Venereol. 2007;21(8):1019-26.

35. Eisen D, Griffiths CE, Ellis CN, Nickoloff BJ, Voorhees JJ. Cyclosporin wash for oral lichen planus. Lancet 1990;335: 5356.

36. Epstein JB. Topical cyclosporine in a bioadhesive for treatment of oral lichenoid mucosal reactions An open label clinical trial. Oral Surg Oral Med Oral Pathol Oral 1996;82:532-6.

37.   Azana JM, Misa RF, Boixeda JP, Ledo A. Topical cyclosporine for cicatricial pemphigoid. J Am Acad Dermatol 1993;28:134–5.

38.   Morrison L, Kratochvil FJ III, Gorman A. An open trial of topical tacrolimus for erosive oral lichen planus. J Am Acad Dermatol 2002; 47:617-20.

39.   Gunther C, Wozel G, Meurer M, Pfeiffer C. Topical tacrolimus treatment for cicatricial pemphigoid. J Am Acad Dermatol 2004;50:325–6.

40.   Sengupta PR. Medical Pharmacology. 1st ed. CBS Publisher 2009; 573-575.

41.   Singhal KC. Essentials of pharmacotherapeutics. 1st ed. CBS Publishers 2007; 11-12.

42.   Sharon, Epstein JB, Inger von Bu "ltzingsl€owen, Scott Drucker, Rinat Tzach & Noam Yarom. Topical immunomodulators for management of oral mucosal conditions, a systematic review. Expert Opin. Emerging Drugs (2011) 16(1):183-202.

43.   Rahul Saxena et al. Immunomodulator A New Horizon: An overview. Journal of Pharmacy Research 2012,5(4),2306-2310.

44.   Panda UN. Textbook of Medicine. 1st ed. CBS Publishers 2000; 107-108.

45.   Hamuryudan V, Ozyazgan Y, Hizli N et al. Azathioprine in Behcet's syndrome: effects on long-term prognosis. Arthritis Rheum 1997; 40: 769–774.

46.   Vivek V, Bindu J Nair. Recurrent Aphthous Stomatitis: Current Concepts in Diagnosis and Management. Journal of Indian Academy of Oral Medicine and Radiology, 2011;23(3):232-236.

47.   Kaushal K et al. Azathioprine for the Treatment of Severe Erosive Oral and Generalized Lichen Planus.Acta Derm Venereol 2001. 378-38.

48.   Malekzad F. Low dose Methotrexate for the treatment of generalized lichen planus.Iran J Dermatol 2011; 14: 131-135.

49.   Neff AG, Turner M, Mutasim DF. Treatment strategies in mucous membrane pemphigoid. Therapeutics and Clinical Risk Management 2008:4(3) 617–626.

50.   Brody HJ, Pirozzi DJ. Benign mucous membrane pemphigoid. Response to therapy with cyclophosphamide. Arch Dermatol 1977;113:1598–9.

51. Mythili MD, Nair SC. Effect of cyclophosphamide pretreatment on hematological indices of Indian Bonnet monkey. Indian J. Pharmacol. 2004; 36: 175-180.

52. Melikoglu M, Fresko I, Mat C et al. Short-term trial of etanercept in Behçet's disease: a double blind, placebo controlled study. J Rheumatol 2005; 32: 98–105.

53. Golan DE. Principles of Pharmacology. The Pathophysiologic Basic of Drug Therapy. 2nd ed. Lippincott 2008; 795-809.

54. Saif SR. Pharmacology Review. 1st ed. CBS Publisher 2005; 99, 846-852.

55. Sugerman PB, Savage NW, Walsh LJ, et al. The pathogenesis of oral lichen planus. Crit Rev Oral Biol Med 2002; 13 (4): 350-65.

56. Spencer-Green G. Etanercept (Enbrel): update on therapeutic use. Ann Rheum Dis 2000 Nov; 59 Suppl. 1: i46-9.

57. Robinson ND, Guitart J. Recalcitrant, recurrent aphthous stomatitis treated with etanercept. Arch Dermatol 2003 Oct; 139 (10): 1259-62.

58. Chiang KY, Abhyankar S, Bridges K, et al. Recombinant human tumor necrosis factor receptor fusion protein as complementary treatment for chronic graft versus-host disease. Transplantation 2002 Feb 27; 73 (4): 665-7.

59. Maender JL, Krishnan RS, Angel TA, et al. Complete resolution of generalized lichen planus after treatment with thalidomide. J Drugs Dermatol 2005 Jan-Feb; 4 (1): 86-8.

60. Haugeberg G, Velken M, Johnson V. Successful treatment of genital ulcers with infliximab in Behçet's disease. Ann Rheum Dis 2004; 63: 744–745.

61. Remicade for Healthcare Professionals". *remicade.com. Archived from* the original*on 2008-07-04.*

62. Rang HP,Dale MM. Rang and dale Pharmacology. 6th ed. Churchill Livingestone Elsevier 2007; 481-488, 538-541.

63. Richar AH, Pamela CC. Lippincott's Illustrated Reviews: Pharmacology. 4th ed. 2009; 489-498.

64. Rebora A, Parodi A, Murialdo G. Basiliximab Is Effective for Erosive Lichen Planus. Arch Dermatol. 2002;138(8):11001101.

65.   A.D. Katsambas, T.M. Lotti European handbook of dermatological treatments 2nd edition, 2003, page 291, ISBN 3-540-00878-0.

66.   Cheng A. Oral Erosive Lichen Planus Treated With Efalizumab. Arch Dermatol/142, 2006 680-82.

67.   Gorouhi F et al. Randomized trial of Pimecrolimus cream versus Triamcinolone acetonide paste in the treatment of oral lichen planus. J Am Acad Dermatol 2007 Nov; 57(5) :806-13.

68.   Mimura MAM,Hirota SK, Sugaya NN, Sanches Jr. JA, Migliari DA. Systemic treatment in severe cases of recurrent aphthous stomatitis: an open trial. Clinics. 2009;64(3):193-8.

69.   Rogers III RS, Seehafer JR, Perry HO. Treatment of cicatricial (benign mucous membrane) pemphigoid with dapsone. J Am Acad Dermatol 1982;6:215–23.

70.   Grinspan D, Blanco GF, Aguero S. Treatment of aphthae with thalidomide. J Am Acad Dermatol 1989; 20: 1060–1063.

71.   Wu Yet al.A randomized double-blind, positive-control trial of topical Thalidomide in erosive oral lichen planus Oral Surg Oral Med Oral Pathol Oral Radiol Endod. 2010 Aug;110(2):188-95.

72.   Shah D, Londhe V, Parikh R. Can levamisole alone maintain the immunity? Int. Jrnl. of pharmacy and pharmaceutical sciences 2011; 3 (2): 161-164.

73.   Barrons RW. Treatment strategies for recurrent oral aphthous ulcers. Am J Helath Syst Pharm 2001; 58: 41–50.

74.   Tai Hyok et al.Levamisole Monotherapy for Oral Lichen Planus. Ann Dermatol Vol. 21, No. 3, 2009.

75.   Lu Sy et al.Dramatic response to Levamisole and low-dose prednisolone in 23 patients with oral lichen planus: a 6-year prospective follow-up study. Oral Surg Oral Med Oral Pathol Oral Radiol Endod 1995;80:705-709.

76.   Xiong C et al. The efficacy of topical intralesional BCGPSN injection in the treatment of erosive oral lichen planus: a randomized controlled trial. J Oral Pathol Med 2009 Aug; 38(7) :551-8.

77.   Zouboulis Ch C, Orfanos CE. Treatment of AdamantiadesBehçet's disease with systemic interferon alfa. Arch Dermatol 1998; 134: 1010–1016.

78.   Haque MF, Meghji S, Nazir R, Harris M. Interferongamma (IFN-gamma) may reverse oral submucous fibrosis. J Oral Pathol Med.2001;30: 12–21.

79.   Fontes V, Machet L, Huttenberger B, Lorette G, Vaillant L.Recurrent aphthous stomatitis: treatment with colchicine.An open trial of 54 cases.Ann Dermatol Venereol 2002; 129:1365– 1369.

80.   Vaibhav D Aher. Herbal medicinal Plants: As an immunomodulator. Nat Prod Chem Res 2017, 5:3.

81.   Singh N, Tailang M, Mehta.A review on herbal plants as immunomodulators. International journal of pharmaceutical sciences and research. E-ISSN: 0975-8232; P-ISSN: 2320-5148.

82.   Chulet R, Pradhan P. A review on rasayana. *Phcog Rev* 2010; 3(6):229e34.

83.   D. Kumar et al.A review of immunomodulators in the Indian traditional health care system.Journal of Microbiology, Immunology and Infection (2012) 45,165e184.

84.   Wagner H In: Hikino H, Farnsworth NR, editors. *Economic andmedicinal plant research*, vol. 1. London: Academic Press; 1984. 113e53.

85.   Blasdell KS, Sharma HM, Tomlinson Jr PF, Wallace RK. Subjective survey, blood chemistry and complete blood profile of subjects taking Maharishi Amrit Kalash (MAK). *FASEB J* 1991;5:A1317.

86.   Rathee P, Chaudhary H, Rathee S, Rathee D, Kumar V. Immunosuppressants: A Review. J The Pharma Innovation.2013, 1 ;(12).

87.   Vaibhav D. Aher; Wahi; Arunkumar: Pharmacological study of Tinospora cordifolia as an Immunomodulator; International Journal of Current Pharmaceutical Research.

88.   Alok, SinghID,Shivani S, Mallika K, Prakash C. Curcumin – Pharmacological Actions And its Role in Oral Submucous Fibrosis: A ReviewJ Clin Diagn Res. 2015 Oct; 9(10): ZE01–ZE03.

89.   Tripathi KD: Essential of Medical Pharmacology.6th edition, JAYPEE Brothers Medical Publisher: 837- 844.

90.   Park's Textbook of Preventive and Social Medicine 21th St. Banarsidas Bhanot Publishers, Prem nagar Jabalpur: year 2011; 421- 443.

91.   Tirtha S.S: The Ayurvedic Encyclopedia. Bayville N.Y.:Ayurvedic Holistic Center Press 1998; 102-103.

92.   Mangaiyarkarasi SP, Manigandan T, Elumalai M, Cholan PK, Kaur RP. Benefits of Aloe vera in dentistry. J Pharm Bioall Sci 2015;7:S255-9.

93.   Moore TE. The M and M's of Aloe vera – Is it for dentistry? J Okla Dent Assoc 2001;91:30-1, 36.

94.   Satoskar RS, Bhandarkar SD, Rege NN. Pharmacology and Pharmacotherauptics (22nd ed), Mumbai, India. Popular Prakashan 2011:819.

95.   Mali AM, Behal R, Gilda SS. Comparative evaluation of 0.1% turmeric mouthwash with 0.2% chlorhexidine gluconate in prevention of plaque and gingivitis: A clinical and microbiological study. J Indian Soc Periodontol 2012;16:386-91.

96.   http://www.Aloeverabenefits.com/index.html

97.   Bagga MB, Jindal S, Chauhan N. Therapeutic effects of Tulsi (Ocimum sanctum Linn) in general and oral health. J Periodontal Med Clin Prac 2016;03: 147-152.

98.   Setty, Arathi R., and Leonard H. Sigal. "Herbal medications commonly used in the practice of rheumatology: mechanisms of action, efficacy, and side effects." In Seminars in arthritis and rheumatism, vol. 34, no. 6, pp. 773-784. Elsevier, 2005.

99.   Pattanayak, Priyabrata, Pritishova Behera, Debajyoti Das, and Sangram K. Panda. "Ocimum sanctum Linn. A reservoir plant for therapeutic applications: An overview." Pharmacognosy reviews 4, no. 7 (2010): 95.

100.   Gowrishankar, Ramadurai, Manish Kumar, Vinay Menon, Sai Mangala Divi, M. Saravanan, P. Magudapathy, B. K. Panigrahi, K. G. M. Nair, and K.

Venkataramaniah. "Trace element studies on Tinospora cordifolia (Menispermaceae), Ocimum sanctum (Lamiaceae), Moringa oleifera (Moringaceae), and Phyllanthus niruri (Euphorbiaceae) using PIXE." Biological trace element research 133, no. 3 (2010): 357-363.

101. Kulshreshtha A, Zacharia AJ, Jarouliya U, Bhadauriya P, Prasad GB, Bisen PS. Spirulina in health care management. *Curr Pharm Biotechnol.* 2008;9(5):400-405.18855693.

102. Ciferri O. Spirulina, the edible microorganism. *Microbiol Rev.* 1983;47(4):551-578.6420655.

103. Ciferri O, Tiboni O. The biochemistry and industrial potential of Spirulina. *Annu Rev Microbiol.* 1985;39:503-526.3933408.

104. Dillon JC, Phuc AP, Dubacq JP. Nutritional value of the alga Spirulina. *World Rev Nutr Diet.* 1995;77:32-46.7732699.

105. Robb-Nicholson C. By the way, doctor. I read that spirulina is the next wonder vitamin. What can you tell me about it? *Harv Womens Health Watch.* 2006;14(3):8.

106. Mulk1BS, DeshpandeP, NagalakshmiV, ChappidiV, Raja lakshmi C.Spirulina and Pentoxyfilline – A Novel Approach for Treatment of Oral Submucous Fibrosis.Journal of Clinical and Diagnostic Research. 2013 Dec, Vol-7(12): 3048-30503048 3048.

107. Mazokopakis EE, Karefilakis CM, Tsartsalis AN, Milkas AN, Ganotakis ES. Acute rhabdomyolysis caused by Spirulina (*Arthrospira platensis*). *Phytomedicine.* 2008;15(6-7):525-527.18434120.

108. Iwasa M, Yamamoto M, Tanaka Y, Kaito M, Adachi Y. Spirulina-associated hepatotoxicity. *Am J Gastroenterol.* 2002;97(12):3212-3213.12492223.

109. Rawn DF, Niedzwiadek B, Lau BP, Saker M. Anatoxin-a and its metabolites in blue-green algae food supplements from Canada and Portugal. *J Food Prot.* 2007;70(3):776-779.

110. Jiang Y, Xie P, Chen J, Liang G. Detection of the hepatotoxic microcystins in 36 kinds of cyanobacteria Spirulina food products in China. *Food Addit Contam Part A Chem Anal Control Expo Risk Assess.* 2008;25(7):885-894.18569007.

111. Wu JF, Pond WG. Amino acid composition and microbial contamination of *Spirulina maxima*, a blue-green alga, grown on the effluent of fermented animal wastes. *Bull Environ Contam Toxicol.* 1981;27(2):151-159.6794684.

112. Lee AN, Werth VP. Activation of autoimmunity following use of immunostimulatory sherbal supplements. *Arch Dermatol.* 2004;140(6):723-727.15210464.

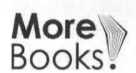
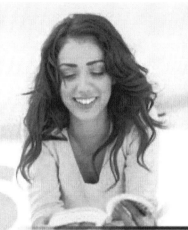 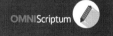

FSC
www.fsc.org

MIX

Papier aus ver-
antwortungsvollen
Quellen
Paper from
responsible sources

FSC® C141904

Druck:
Customized Business Services GmbH
im Auftrag der KNV-Gruppe
Ferdinand-Jühlke-Str. 7
99095 Erfurt